OVERCOMING STROKE

The 5 Keys to Victory

VALERIE L. GREENE

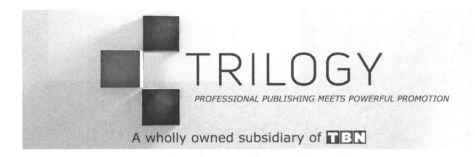

TRILOGY
PROFESSIONAL PUBLISHING MEETS POWERFUL PROMOTION

A wholly owned subsidiary of TBN

Overcoming Stroke
Trilogy Christian Publishers
A Wholly Owned Subsidiary of Trinity Broadcasting Network
2442 Michelle Drive
Tustin, CA 92780
For information, address Trilogy Christian Publishing
Rights Department, 2442 Michelle Drive, Tustin, Ca 92780.
Trilogy Christian Publishing/ TBN and colophon are trademarks of Trinity Broadcasting Network.
For information about special discounts for bulk purchases, please contact Trilogy Christian Publishing.
Manufactured in the United States of America

10 9 8 7 6 5 4 3 2 1
Library of Congress Cataloging-in-Publication Data is available.
ISBN: 978-1-63769-822-8
ISBN: 978-1-63769-823-5

DEDICATION

To my precious mother who by example taught me how to walk by faith, and show others compassion, kindness, & love.

I love you, Mom.

Valerie

In Special Honor of Jan Crouch
Co-Founder of TBN
(Trinity Broadcasting Network)

Died of a massive stroke
May 31, 2016
Orlando, FL

Her stroke led me to TBN so the world
could hear the good news!

FOREWORD

Working with Valerie Greene has been, is always, a blessed opportunity. Her perspective and drive are true. Her mission is to help stroke survivors, and she brings experience, resources, and knowledge to the table.

Recovering from stroke herself, she knows what it's like, in all stages. Her compassion added to her knowledge makes it easy to trust her. Val originally designed the B-Center, a healing center for stroke survivors. When obstacles came into view, she never gave up.

So, when she started coaching, it was years of thinking of every aspect of how to help others that got her there. This book is one more way she's trying to help every person she can. Trust is perhaps the biggest factor when choosing a coach, a healing modality, or a healing product. You will not find a more trustworthy person to invest time and energy with than Valerie Greene. Her purpose is to help stroke survivors and she has dedicated her life to it.

She's taken her brilliance and kindness and focused it on stroke prevention and recovery. Because she spent years seeking natural methods for her own healing and the proper guidance, she wants to help show others the way. Sheer determination and her belief led to her walking, talking, functioning. She took her vibrancy and kept going – learning how to further heal, what more to know, to discover, to relate to healing. Valerie is bright, articulate, and relatable. She has business acumen and a sense of order and organization. But what will strike you when you meet her is her compassion, her keen listening skills, her caring. Don't hesitate to contact her for guidance. As you will see from this book, she has formulated a plan that works.

Gay Lacy, LMT

ACKNOWLEDGMENTS

My deepest gratitude to all the dear people that God has placed in my life throughout my journey to help and uplift me. We are not meant to go through life trying to do everything ourselves - we need one another. I am so thankful for the outpouring of love and generosity from everyone – family, friends, healthcare providers, business associates and so many more for sharing their time, talents, and blessings with me. It has not gone unnoticed. I am humbled and forever grateful.

Thank you to my dear mother who has always kept me lifted in prayer. Thank you, Mom, for giving me the greatest gift of all - my faith and trust in Jesus Christ as my Savior and Messiah. Having the comfort of knowing He is in control and that no matter what He is always with me and will never leave me is priceless. I am comforted with a peace that passes all understanding.

PROLOGUE

To all my fellow stroke warriors. You have survived one of the most devastating health challenges to the human body. That means you are here for a reason and you have a purpose. Life is not over!

There is no way around the fact that having a stroke changes your life, but it doesn't need to be the end of living. I was told I may never walk or talk again but look at me now! Sadly, these types of bleak forecasts are more common than not. I've always said it would be better to say nothing or to simply say, *"I don't know"* than to diminish someone's hope. Because truthfully, no one knows, but God.

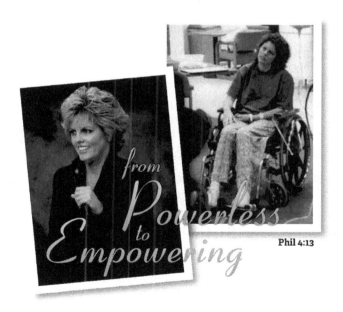

Phil 4:13

I'm going to help you discover what I learned to ignite and accelerate the healing process that resulted in my own recovery from a massive stroke. I have been where you are and walked in your shoes. If someone had told me the things that I am going to share with you in this book, I could have been spared years of searching and suffering. I've seen how the human body regenerates from the worst injuries when given the right things.

There are good and bad products, technologies, and therapies. Knowing which ones to use correctly can make all the difference. I like to think of it as selecting the right ingredients for a recipe, or materials to build a house. You need specific items used properly to produce the best outcome.

Like many of you, I was determined to find answers and solutions. I spent years and a small fortune traveling all around the world searching and trying every therapy, modality, and unique protocols. I'm sure you will understand when I say that I was willing to try anything. Then one day I realized that the answers had been near me all along. They were so simple I had overlooked them. I was expecting some expensive treatment from a faraway place provided by a guru to make the difference. Instead, I decided to look within and ask my maker - consult my creator. No different than going directly to a manufacturer for a question regarding one of their products. You wouldn't take your computer to the gas station for repairs. We have a creator that designed us with the ability to heal. So, why not ask for help? Made sense to me. It wasn't an instant revelation, but over time it was as if my eyes were being opened to see clearly. And, then it all came together.

Lean in for this, because I'm going to give you a golden clue ... the things we will die without are the key ingredients that our bodies need to heal — healthy water, oxygen, and good blood flow. The secret is knowing how best to accomplish this and what products and therapies to use.

This book is intended to provide an overview of my personal formula that has made a dramatic difference in my personal recovery and on-going well-being.

INTRODUCTION

Like so many of us, I never imagined my health being challenged with a life-altering illness. Yet, at age thirty-one I suffered two strokes that nearly ended my life. As I cried out for a drink of water in the Emergency Room, I was told that I could not have anything to drink because I was suffering a neurological event. But my body knew what they didn't – I was chronically dehydrated.

While the culprit was a blood clot that occluded the basilar artery in my brain stem, (95% fatal) the origin was never determined. For years the question stumped the medical community - "Why would a healthy young woman suffer a massive stroke with no known history of any health issues?"

Through many years of conventional and natural therapies, I was blessed with good guidance and wisdom to act on what I was taught. Without discovering how the body repairs and heals itself, coupled with God's amazing grace, I would not be here today.

This book reveals the secrets that I discovered throughout my journey that we all seem to take for granted and often miss. May you be enlightened, empowered and encouraged to take action.

TABLE OF CONTENTS

THE 5 KEYS TO VICTORY

STROKE 101

Strokes affect approximately 33 million people world-wide. They strike at random and can target anyone: young, old, men, women, even children. A stroke, also known as a transient ischemic attack (TIA), happens when there is an instantaneous interruption of blood and, consequently, oxygen to the brain. Even when caught and treated quickly, strokes still cause some serious long-term problems.

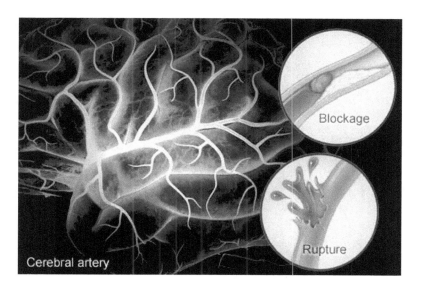

There are two different main types of strokes that we experience today. The first is the hemorrhagic stroke. This stroke is when a blood vessel ruptures causing internal bleeding. This type of stroke can be due to high blood pressure, but aneurysms and malformation in your arteries can also cause this to happen. The second type of stroke is the ischemic stroke, the most common; 85 percent of all strokes are ischemic (as was mine). It is caused by a blood clot depriving the brain of oxygen and nutrients. You can also experience what is often called a mini-stroke, where you have blood clots, but they don't block the path of the blood for long, and there is usually no permanent damage.

WHO THIS IS FOR?

This is for anyone who has suffered a stroke and wants to overcome the emotional and physical devastation of a stroke and live a life of health, happiness, and hope. Whether you've been struggling for years or just had a stroke, either way, this is for you!

In this book you will discover …

- How to turn your life around and get back to having a life filled with energy and vitality.

- How to get rid of that wheelchair, or cane, and walk without assistance.

- How to recover from a stroke without spending the rest of your life going to rehab or traveling far away to undergo experimental treatments or surgeries.

- How to get restful sleep, even if you've been tossing and turning for months, to waking up feeling refreshed and ready for a new day filled with endless possibilities!

- How to do all this without prescription drugs, shots, surgeries, experimental, or expensive treatments.

LET'S BE CLEAR

- This is not a silver bullet "quick fix."

- This is not a "do nothing, get better."

- You need to want to overcome and be ready to take action!

DOES THIS SOUND LIKE YOU?

- Do you start off every day wondering ... Now what?

- Is your mind reeling with questions wondering if you're ever going to get better?

- Are you TERRIFIED of having another stroke?

- Do you secretly have thoughts of not going on?

- Do you see everyone doing things that you can no longer do? – Like riding a bike, walking without assistance, driving a car?

- Are you working tirelessly at rehab and seeing little to no results?

- Do you feel overwhelmed and exhausted?

- Do you feel like there is a ceiling on your recovery?

If any of that sounds like you then I have good news –
None of those things are the real problem.
Those are just the symptoms.

THE REAL PROBLEM

You haven't used the right keys

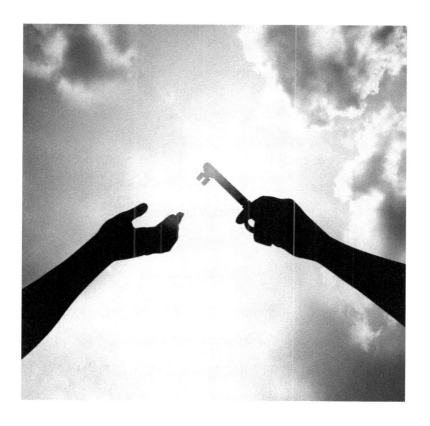

ONCE YOU USE THE RIGHT KEYS...

- You will see light at the end of the tunnel.

- You will be encouraged and have hope.

- You can thrive - not just survive!

- No more endless trips to rehab to do countless exercises or researching the internet for the latest trial treatment. You can relax and let your body begin to heal naturally.

- Clear your brain fog, sleep better, have more energy, destroy depression, and let your body begin to heal. All the years of frustration that you've gone through are going to pay off because your body will finally be working for you instead of against you.

- You're going to finally start to see progress and feel great.

BUSTING MYTHS & MISCONCEPTIONS

Most everything out there is based on conventional wisdom that tells us ...

- The most recovery only occurs in the first six months.
- The brain doesn't recover.
- You need to be on medications the rest of your life.

It is frustrating that these things are still being told to survivors and their families. No wonder people are so depleted of hope. Hope is essential for recovery. I literally had to force myself to avoid negative input and draw to messages of hope. When I heard a negative prediction or comment I simply told myself to cancel it. You have to be in control of what you allow to enter your mind & spirit. Unfortunately, there will always be naysayers (often those closest to you). I had well-meaning friends tell me I was living in denial - that I wasn't accepting reality. To which I always replied that I'd rather aim for something really big and fail than to think small and succeed. So, the next time someone tells you their small vision of your outcome - cancel that and tell yourself ... Yes, I can and WILL overcome!

Negative messages are always going to be around. It's up to us to choose to tune out them out and change the channel or narrative and envision the best. What you hear in your spirit will override what you see in the natural. We constantly have to fight our nature to be drawn to bad news or the unknown. I've always found it interesting that weather meteorologists say there is a 50 percent chance of rain vs saying there is a 50 percent chance of sunshine. The odds are equal, so why not choose the most favorable outcome?

As you probably figured by now, I'm an optimist. I prefer to see the glass half full. While I have a scientific mind, I am a visionary choosing to see the best. Bottom line, I know God is in control, so I have peace in the midst of the storm.

DISCOVERING THE KEYS TO VICTORY

Just like building a house requires a contractor, plan, and materials, overcoming a stroke is no different - you need good guidance, a road map, and the right tools. I've seen so many people run from one thing to the next trying to find answers and help. I did the same thing. It's exhausting and often futile. So, learn from me – your body will heal when you give it the right things; be consistent and allow time for the transformation to take place. You wouldn't expect a woman to give birth after only a few months of being pregnant. Anything worthwhile takes time. I get it, you want to heal fast. I was no different. Having a plan and doing the right things will certainly move you faster and in the right direction, it just won't be overnight. Slow and steady is the winning ticket. Remember, the turtle won the race.

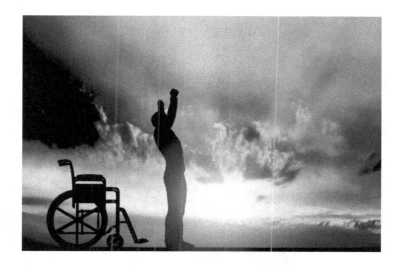

YOUR VICTORY AWAITS!

Looking back on my own recovery it felt like forever. But as many people tell me, the progress and transformation were remarkable to watch. It will surprise you to know how many people are watching you. After years of shopping in Publix, a lady in the bakery decided to tell me how much she and her co-workers were inspired by watching my recovery. They shared memories of the times when I would come in the store with my walker and do "cart therapy." That was my own version of therapy to re-learn how to walk by pushing a grocery cart. It always made me feel good to be in public doing "normal" things. It was therapeutic for both my body and mind.

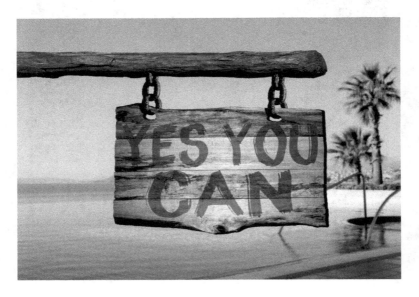

A SOLID FOUNDATION

For a successful recovery you must begin with a solid foundation.

The first key that I will be sharing is perhaps the most important of all – the platform on which the success of everything else is determined – your mindset represents your foundation.

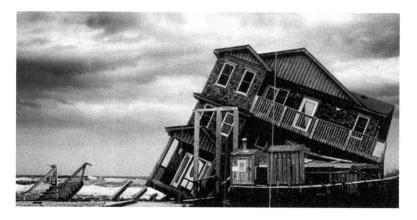

I cannot stress the importance of your mindset and building on a solid foundation. No matter how bleak things may appear, you've got to see yourself overcoming. The only way that this is possible is to first believe that you can.

During my recovery, I converted my guest room into a

workout space with a treadmill facing a wall covered with images of things I would like to see myself doing. I'd spend hours cutting out pictures from magazines and putting them on the wall. It was my vision board. There were images of a woman riding a horse; walking in a marathon; speaking before a large audience; even driving a Mercedes. When friends would stop by, I could almost hear their thoughts of pity thinking I would probably never do any of these things.

But, by the grace of God I have done them all. Because I believed, and then constantly saw myself doing what I was told I couldn't; walking unassisted, driving a nice car, and being a voice for my fellow survivors. I allowed my mind to drown out the negative voices that were telling me differently.

Recovery requires engaging your mind, body, and spirit. You need all three. Your foundation is the framework that holds everything up. So, be careful what you let in. You can catch a thought just like you can catch a cold.

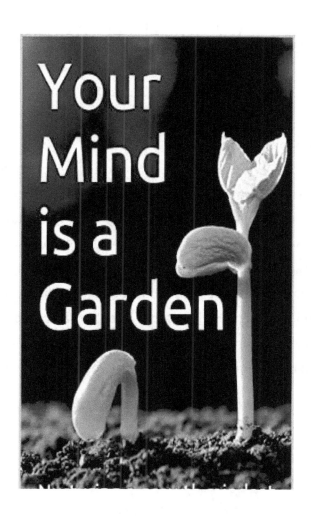

KEY #1

RENEW YOUR MIND

The Master Key

Everything begins in our mind as a thought or image. What we think, see, and believe transcend to the rest of our body. You've probably heard … "Where the mind goes, the body will follow," or the verse ... "As a man thinks, so is he." A common saying is … "Thoughts become things." This awareness is becoming more mainstream as it has been studied and found to have profound outcomes. No longer is it just a thought, theory or belief. It is scientifically proven. Your mind is your control center and battlefield. Once you get this, you will be careful as to who and what you will allow in.

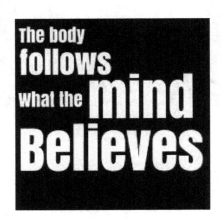

Our mindset is one of the most useful powers we possess. What we think, envision or believe can create success or failure, happiness or unhappiness, opportunities or obstacles. Pay attention to what you're telling yourself or allowing others to tell you.

Every day we make choices to trust in things we cannot see or understand. We trust there is air even though we can't see it. We trust gravity even though we don't fully understand it. Why should trusting God be any different? This is why I encourage everyone to draw close to positive input that is faith based so we can be better equipped to guard our heart and mind against the barrage of negativity we live amongst. Whether by reading or hearing, we need to saturate our mind with things that uplift, inspire, and encourage us to be all we can be! Just like our bodies need food, so do our souls. And the quality of what we put in will determine what we produce. Plant an apple seed; you will produce an apple tree.

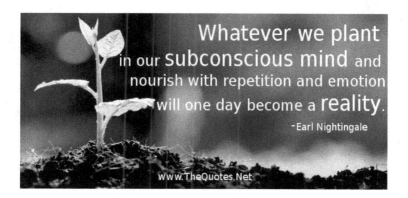

Whatever we plant in our subconscious mind and nourish with repetition and emotion will one day become a reality.

-Earl Nightingale

www.TheQuotes.Net

My heritage has a long line of faith believers and prayer warriors. I grew up hearing that I was a child of God, and He would never leave or forsake me. So, even when I would get lonely or scared, it would pass when I remembered I was never alone and was safe in the palm of God's hands. How reassuring it was, and still is, to know that even when I don't understand things, or like the situation, God is with me and has a purpose for everything. My faith grew stronger through my stroke and became my anchor of hope. It wasn't always easy, but I learned to let go and trust God. Ever since, I have a peace that passes all understanding that keeps me grounded and has become my compass.

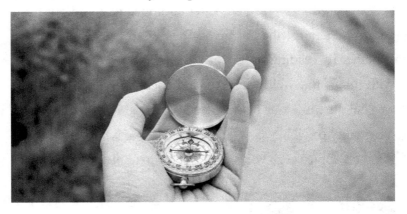

I know it is easy to get discouraged when you can't see a way. This is when you have to make a decision to accept things by faith. You can overcome any obstacle with the faith of a mustard seed. So, rather than tell God how big your mountain is, tell your mountain how big your God is! Don't rely on emotions or feelings. They can deceive and mislead us. Wake up expecting something great. Often, it's not the storms that defeat us, but how we choose to respond.

Bitter or Better

WHICH PATH WILL YOU CHOOSE?

YOUR LIFE IS BEING STEERED – KNOW WHO IS AT THE WHEEL

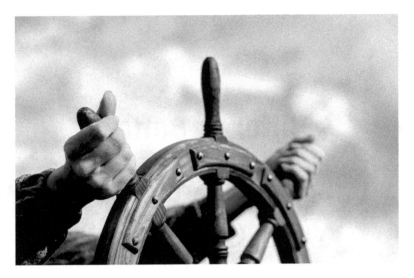

7 Key Principles

1. The body will follow where the mind goes.

2. Be transformed by the renewing of your mind Rom. 12:2 (NIV)

3. As a man thinks, so is he. Prov. 23:7

4. Whether you believe you CAN or CAN'T – You're RIGHT!

5. You have to make your mind up that you CAN and WILL overcome!

6. Thoughts DO become things.

7. Expect restoration! Expect healing!

KEY#2

KNOW WHAT LIES BENEATH

Just like the Titanic was sunk by an iceberg because they were unaware of what was below the surface, our bodies are the same. Stroke is just the result. Something was underlying that triggered it. You MUST become aware so you can address the root cause. Otherwise, you are setting yourself for another stroke and more health issues. The good news is that most of the time the answers are simpler than we expect and can provide great relief and even reverse damages.

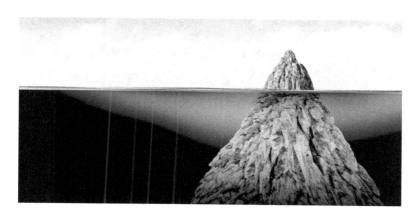

You First Have to be Aware of a Problem

Before You Can Fix It

To understand the cause, we first need to look under the hood, so to speak and examine the elements that our bodies require to keep everything moving efficiently and strong. How well is your blood circulation; your oxygen content and the quality of your drinking water will determine your body's overall performance. Just like a car needs gas, water, and oil to perform, our bodies need basic key essentials to function optimally and the keys to start them.

> **85% of all strokes are caused by a blockage. Blockages slow the flow of blood, oxygen and water – like a train wreck waiting to happen.**

I'm as guilty as anyone for not seeing the forest for the trees. But once I get quite and listen to the still voice within me, my fears fade away and I receive peace. I understand that God brings people in our life to help lead us to the "water" and then it's up to us to drink. We have to do our part.

KEY#3

THE INTEGRATIVE APPROACH

Your Secret Weapons

Throughout my journey I have discovered there are re-markable technologies and therapies to help accelerate our body's own natural healing ability. I refer to them as "Secret Weapons." Working together is the key.

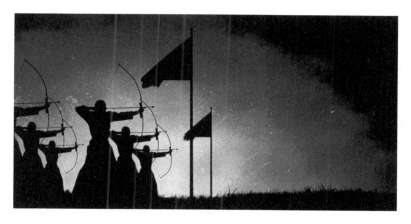

In this section, I will be sharing the key modalities and therapies I personally used to accelerate my recovery and continue to use for my on-going health and wellness. Keep

in mind that while each of us is unique, there are basic prin-
ciples by which we heal. Results will vary but will only oc-
cur when we decide to take action.

HAVING THE RIGHT TOOLS MATTERS!

We Learn from Either Mentors or Mistakes

Aside from a miracle (which does and can happen) you need tools. A stroke is an enormous battle of the mind, spirit, and body. Having the right guidance and tools can change things faster & easier.

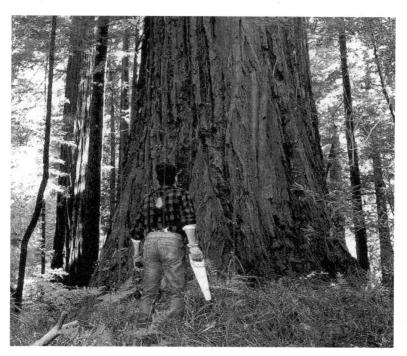

Oxygen Therapy

When part of your brain isn't getting enough blood, that means it isn't getting enough oxygen. The longer your brain goes without oxygen, the more damage a stroke can do. Shortly after my stroke, I was referred to a renowned physician in South Florida who was a pioneer in oxygen therapy. He used Hyperbaric Oxygen Therapy (HBOT) as a means to restore the depleted oxygen that occurs in the brain following a stroke. He explained how this therapy "wakes up" the stunned cells that are assumed dead. He went on to say - that while some brain cells do die, many are stunned and can be restored. This was so encouraging and turned out true in my case.

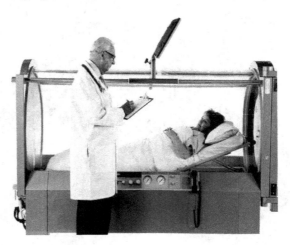

According to the Mayo Clinic, the theory behind using HBOT for stroke is that increasing the supply of oxygen to the parts of the brain affected by stroke may lessen brain swelling and protect brain cells, reducing the extent of irreversible brain damage and leading to better outcomes.

WHAT IS HYPERBARIC OXYGEN THERAPY (HBOT)?

Hyperbaric Oxygen Therapy (HBOT) is a noninvasive and painless treatment used for restoring oxygen to tissues that have been damaged by oxygen deprivation. Using pure oxygen under increased pressure, the body's natural ability to heal from traumas, diseases and other afflictions is enhanced – and in many cases, is accelerated.

The resistance that is common in the United States does not exist in other parts of the world, where HBOT is used to treat more than 73 medical conditions, including stroke. It is widely practiced in the United Kingdom, Europe, Russia, South America, and Asia.

In a Hyperbaric Oxygen Therapy chamber, the air pressure is increased two to three times higher than normal air pressure. Under these conditions, your lungs can gather much more oxygen than would be possible breathing pure oxygen at normal air pressure. When your blood carries this extra oxygen throughout your body, this helps fight bacteria and stimulate the release of substances called growth factors and stem cells, which promote healing.

I can attest that all my therapies were accelerated by having HBOT. I underwent thirty sessions (aka dives) in my first round and started seeing visible results. It was relaxing as I would watch movies or sleep.

Always do your research on the facility and equipment being used. There are only a couple of mono chambers that I personally would ever use - Sechrist is my first choice.

WATER

Throughout my recovery, I learned a great deal about water from some of the best teachers in the world. It was fascinating and revealed many mysteries. Water is much more than most of us think. It is the foundation for wellness and essential to stroke recovery. I'm going to share some of what I discovered so you will better understand its vital role in our health and healing.

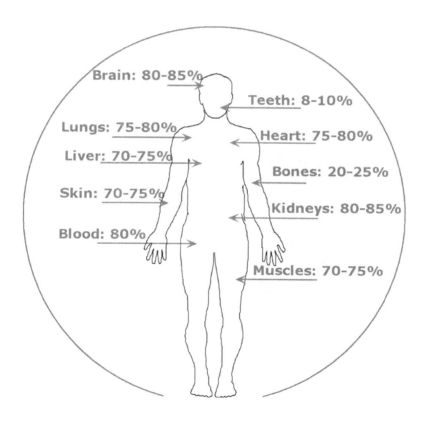

"Drinking the right water, not just any water, is critical for your health and prevention of disease. This is true, now more than ever."

- Horst S. Filtzer, MD
F.A.C.S. Former Chief of Surgery,
Cambridge Hospital, Harvard Medical School

Without Water We Will Die

Our brain is 85 percent water. It is the first organ that loses water and becomes dehydrated. This accounts for brain fog, headaches and not being able to think clearly. When there isn't enough water available to your brain, your brain basically shuts down to conserve energy.

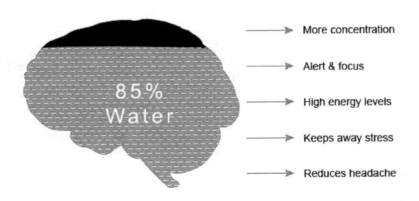

85% Water

More concentration

Alert & focus

High energy levels

Keeps away stress

Reduces headache

So, if our brains are mostly water, then it is only logical that lack of water can cause the brain some real problems. Alterations in the balance of brain water contribute significantly to morbidity and death associated with many common neurological disorders including head trauma, stroke, tumors, infections, and metabolic disorders.

All of These Neurological Conditions Can Be Triggered by a Lack of Hydration in the Brain:

DEHYDRATION OF THE BRAIN

- Alzheimer's disease
- Seizures
- Allergies
- Depression
- Anxiety
- Parkinson's
- Schizophrenia
- Stroke
- Acidosis
- Autism
- Alcoholism
- Behavioral disorders
- Personality disorders
- Coma
- Asperger's

Most Common Signs of Dehydration:

- Thirst
- Headache
- Nausea
- Dry Skin
- Dark Colored Urine
- Fatigue & Weakness
- Head Rushes
- Dizziness
- Cramps
- Dry Mouth
- Constipation
- Irritability

Could Healthy Water Prevent Strokes?

At least once a day I am asked, "What is the number one thing you would do to prevent a stroke?" And, I always say – "You're going to think it's too simple, but the truth is to stay hydrated with fresh clean water."

All Water is Not Equal –
Choose Your Water Wisely

Most of us do not reach for water as a beverage of choice for good reason – it usually doesn't taste or smell good. This could be why – most of our drinking water is tap water and tap water has been shown to be contaminated with an array of chemicals, pesticides, pharmaceuticals and even fecal matter. It is disgusting and dangerous. And it will never benefit brain recovery, in fact it could cause more damage. Bottled water is not much better as most has been proven to be nothing more than slightly filtered tap water. Plus, most of the toxic chemicals in the plastic leach into the water after sitting in a hot warehouse or delivery truck. It is also dead and clunky – meaning the H20 water molecule has so much stuff attached to it that it becomes too large to penetrate the cell membrane, leaving it stuck in your stomach. That's why you get bloated or feel the water sloshing in your stomach. The solution is to drink water that is reduced into microclusters. This means that the water molecule is tiny enough to penetrate the cell wall and cross the blood-brain barrier (BBB).

Cellular Hydration

Water is intended to enter our cells to carry nutrients in and flush out toxins. However, as mentioned earlier, most water is contaminated with an array of substances attached to it, so it becomes too large to penetrate the cell membrane or cross the blood brain barrier. Think of it like trying to throw a bowling ball through a chain link fence versus a handful of BBs.

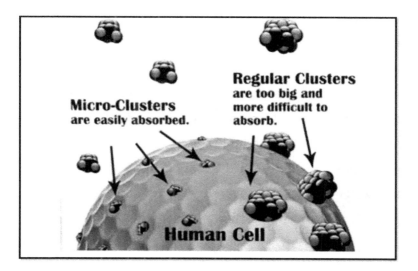

Where do you find micro-clustered water?

There are a few "blue-zones" in the world where this water has been found. But most of us aren't able to fly to the Himalayan mountains for a drink of it. So, over one hundred scientists from around the world studied these waters, and the Japanese invented an electrolysis /ionizer to replicate it. In Japan, this machine it is a certified medical device used in many hospitals and clinics where it is touted as "miracle water." Fortunately, these devices are available worldwide, so from your kitchen sink you can turn ordinary tap water into active "living" water that has an extra electron to boost energy and brain activity, as opposed to "dead" water that washes over your cells leaving you dehydrated. Fresh clean water is vital to your recovery and drinking the right kind of water is imperative. The technology used to produce this water requires high quality components and will generally cost more. Do not compromise when it comes to your health, or you will pay a much higher price later. Just beware there are a lot of machines on the market that claim to produce this water. But as I discovered, very few use superior components and are successful at maintaining a quality output. Most will start off showing good readings but then within months you could be consuming contaminated water as a result of inferior parts and/or design flaws. Worse, you may never realize it.

The (3) main things you want your drinking water to have:

1. A high pH (9.5) - Alkaline

2. A high negative ORP (-300 or greater) - Oxygenated

3. Micro-clustered molecules to pass the Blood-Brain Barrier & cell membrane

NOTE: <u>Not all water can be converted into ionized water.</u> Distilled water products, as well as reverse osmosis (RO) water, CANNOT respond to electrolysis nor can the effect of the separation of the alkaline and acid component be done since both waters lack minerals for the ionization process.

In order to receive the most benefit, be sure to have an experienced person guide you on the selection, installation, and usage. The only water I drink is recognized throughout the world as the gold standard of ionization and the most powerful water on the planet. Known as Kangen water it is endorsed by one of the world's foremost gastroenterologists in addition to thousands of other physicians.

Something as simple as changing the water you drink could change your life.

Water Terms to Know

pH

The term pH stands for "potential Hydrogen." The basic pH chart ranges from 0-14 with 7 being neutral. When your pH is out of the normal range, it opens the doors for disease and sickness. Acidic conditions cause effects at the cellular level and lead to degenerative diseases.

Hexagonal

It is proven that the existence of a specific water structure, known as hexagonal water, is present in various parts of the world. This water is known for its healing and beneficial effects.

Oxidation Reduction Potential (ORP)

ORP is a measurement of oxidized contaminants and the electrical charge in water. The O = Oxidizing and R = Reducing. An ORP meter measures the electrical charge of the water being tested. If it reads (+) positive, it's acidic and is oxidizing. If the meter reads (-) negative, it is alkaline and is an antioxidant. The higher the negative charge the greater the antioxidant potential of the water. Ninety-eight percent of all bottled water and tap water tested for ORP show very high positive charge (number) and acidity.

Ionized Water

Ionized water is drinking water that has undergone a process known as ionization. Essentially, this process separates the acid and alkaline components found in H2O. When successfully ionized, this type of drinking water can help enhance the ability of the blood to carry oxygen and also assist in neutralizing free radicals in the bloodstream. **Not all types of water can be converted into ionized water**. Distilled water products, as well as reverse osmosis (RO) water, cannot respond to electrolysis nor can the effect of the separation of the alkaline and acid component be done since both waters lack minerals for the ionization process.

The Origin of Ionized Water

When studying the history of alkaline water ionization, all roads lead to Hunza of the Himalaya located in Pakistan. The Hunza people are the most studied tribe in the world for their longevity and lack of disease. They live to be over 120-145 and never have any diseases like cancer, diabetes, or strokes. When asked why this is, they credit it to their water. Advanced technology now allows us to reproduce this type of water. Technology in this case has brought the benefits of glacial waters to our homes to aid us in our quest for health and anti-aging.

Nattokinase

A Natural Blood Thinner used for Stroke Prevention & Recovery

Nattokinase is an enzyme that is extracted from a popular Japanese food called natto. It has been used for hundreds of years to thin the blood and help break up blood clots.

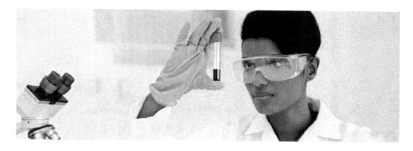

Studies have found that Nattokinase can significantly reduce the increase in fibrinogen seen after a stroke and the severity of a stroke. It also has been found to have a neuroprotective role because of its ability to reduce the clumping together of cells called platelets that help your body form clots, as well as by preventing injured cells from dying.

Following my stroke, I wanted a natural alternative to the traditional pharmaceutical drugs normally used to thin the blood, especially after learning about all the side effects. After consulting with my physician, I made a personal decision to wean off the drug blood thinner that I had been taking and gradually replace it with Nattokinase. It has been nearly thirty years since my stroke, and my blood viscosity is excellent.

Always consult your healthcare provider before making any changes.

MICRO-CIRCULATION

Micro-circulation refers to blood flow in the tiniest blood vessels in the body - the capillaries. Our blood circulation is the key to the body's ability for prevention, healing, recovery and regeneration processes. It is the engine that keeps us going. The heart pumps blood through the main arteries, but it relies on the additional power of the autonomous pumping motion of the micro vessels known as vasomotion. It is these very small vessels that reach the most remote parts of our body. These tiny vessels make up 74 percent of our vascular system. If placed end-to-end, they would extend more than 74,000 miles.

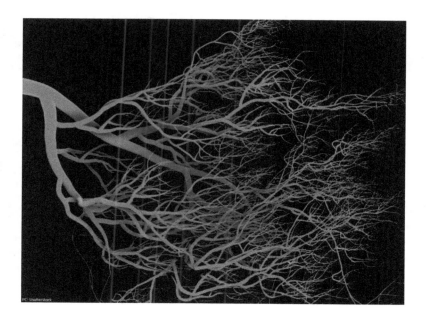

PC: Shutterstock

Like millions of hair-like branches, the capillaries make up most of our blood supply running through our entire body, organs, and bones. So why don't we ever hear about these tiny micro vessels? I believe it's because there is not much that can be done with them. They are two-thirds the size of a strand of hair. Much too small to operate on or treat. Just think if a blockage has been building in the capillaries for a long time, we have no way of knowing until it's too late. Perhaps that's why a stroke is so sudden. The good news is through advanced technology we can address this at the molecular level to restore healthy blood flow and provide both prevention and regeneration.

A Technology That Helps the Body Heal Itself Faster

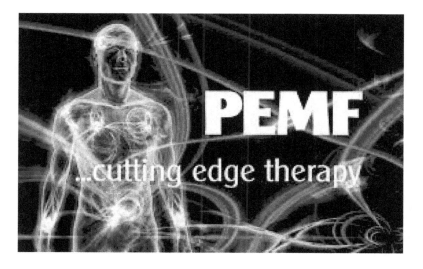

Referred to as "The Silent Healer," pulsed electromagnetic field therapy (PEMF) has been an FDA approved form of treatment for almost forty years. There are many different kinds of PEMF devices. I was treated by several types. Some are designed for clinical use for specific uses and purposes that offer stronger intensities, but the biggest difference is usually found in the wave patterns. Most are administered by a health care professional and could cost as much as a car. Then I discovered one that offered a unique patented wave form (NASA actually chose) that was producing remarkable results, and I could easily use it in the comfort of my home or take it with me when I traveled. Funny thing, when a friend called to tell me about it, he asked if I had BEMER, to which I replied, "No, I drive a Mercedes."

WHAT IS PEMF THERAPY

How Can It Help You?

PEMF stands for Pulsed Electromagnetic Field. PEMF therapy works by recreating the Earth's magnetic fields, which are critical to human life at a cellular level. Pulsating magnetic field generators are now recreated inside NASA spaceships to help maintain optimal health in astronauts and reduce sickness and lack of energy upon re-entering Earth's gravity. Here on Earth, PEMF therapy has seen positive results for individuals suffering from pain or recovering from injury, as well as those with anxiety or depression, or seeking healthier aging. PEMF therapy devices deliver waves in an organized sequence at specific frequencies set to a certain pulse.

There are many PEMF devices vying to be the most effective. Like any technology you need to be careful to select the one best shown to produce positive results and to be safe. One of the devices that I use is a medical device from Germany that has been used in hospitals and clinics around the world for many years. It has a patented signal that targets the micro vessels and increases blood flow and vasomotion. When I first tried it, I didn't recognize any benefit. However, when I loaned it to a friend to use for a week, I felt the difference and had to ask for it back. Since, it has been years since I've gone a day without it, as it's part of my daily routine. Using it daily I find that my energy increases, my hip pain melts away, and I sleep deeply and soundly.

Benefits of Regular Use

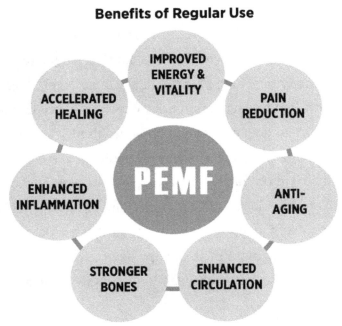

ALSO...
Increased Blood Oxygen Content, Faster Recovery, Strengthened Immune System, and Restored Joints and Muscles

PEMF SIDE EFFECTS

Decades of studies have been made on the positive influence of PEMF on many different ailments. These studies have found PEMF to be beneficial to both humans and animals with no adverse side effects. It is drug-free and non-invasive.

PEMF VS EMF

A common cause of confusion regarding Pulsed Electromagnetic Field Therapy is that it is associated with the harmful Electromagnetic Fields (EMFs) that are present within the environment. However, the pulsed electromagnetic fields differ from the harmful electromagnetic fields in several ways.

Pulsed electromagnetic fields (PEMF) contribute to the healing and improvement of the health of both humans and animals. It is a technology that has been used internationally for several decades to help reverse those imbalances caused by harmful electromagnetic fields by delivering beneficial frequencies to your body. It accomplishes this by sending a pulsing electromagnetic field that stimulates and energizes the cells within your body. Your body takes this energy and then uses it for its natural self-healing functions. Most PEMF devices use low frequencies and long wavelengths, ranging from 1 to 10,000 Hertz, and do not produce any heating action. In comparison, a microwave, which produces harmful EMFs, can use frequencies in the range of 100,000,000 Hertz. Research has shown that pulsed electromagnetic fields in low frequency and intensity can result in an increase of oxygenation to the blood, improve the body's circulation and enhance cell metabolism. Magnetic frequencies help to regulate several processes of the human body. In fact, our bodies even produce their own magnetic fields. However, when artificial and harmful electromagnetic fields enter your body, such as those from cell phone service or power lines, they can disrupt the way your body naturally works, creating an imbalance. I learned this the hard way as both my cats received a death sentence after discovering they had liver cancer. The veterinarians suggested they must have been exposed to something environmental as it was very unusual to see two healthy indoor cats get the exact cancer at the same time. So, as with anything, I began to research for a remedy in hopes to save my dear pets, and myself. It was too late for my precious fur babies, and time was of the essence for me as I was already experiencing the effects of the powerful radiation being emitted from the dozens of cell towers installed on the rooftop of the building where I lived. I knew little about the dangers of EMF exposure and thought it just affected electrosensitive people. So, when this was brought to my attention by my cats' cancer, it made me rethink. After talking with EMF experts, they all told me about products that would help shield the radiation from one or two cell tower transmitters, but unfortunately, not with as many as were on my roof. Cell towers should be a minimum of 400 meters away to be considered safe. (approx. 1,300 feet). A nine-story building is less than 100 feet high. Far too close. Bottomline, nothing would protect me from the abundance of radiation blasting from so many cell transmitters 24/7. Among a multitude of health issues, it has been shown to destroy your DNA and myelin sheath protecting your brain opening the door to a host of neurological issues from memory loss to stroke. Not to mention all the cancer claims. So, I moved from the home I loved. I'm sharing this with you in hopes that you will learn from my experience and explore this topic with seriousness as it can have a huge impact on your recovery and well-being. Sadly, many people dismiss what they cannot see, but just like with carbon monoxide, it is an invisible killer. Learn how to protect yourself @ www.Memon.eu

The International Agency for Research on Cancer, classified radiofrequency EMF as a class 2B carcinogen. European studies show symptoms most commonly reported from people exposed to EMFs: headaches, confusion, cardiac arrhythmias, fibrillations, ear ringing, anxiety, depression, autism, ADD, ADHD etc.

CASE STUDY #1

BETH. MASSIVE STROKE. AGE 35

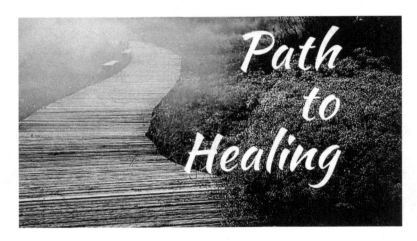

When Beth first came to me, she complained of leg and hip pain, low energy, memory problems, brain fog, and depression. I put together a protocol for her recovery. In just three months of working with Beth, she said she was astounded that after eleven years her body could heal. Her speech improved. She didn't suffer her usual aches and pains; her energy was increased; brain fog and depression diminished. Both her body and mind shifted and now she has a path to follow.

GUT-BRAIN CONNECTION

Stroke Recovery Begins in The Gut

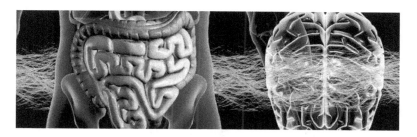

The gut is considered to be our "second brain" and influences the way our brain functions to a large extent through neurotransmitter productions. If the tight junctions (barrier in the gut to protect against toxins leaking into the bloodstream) aren't functioning properly, the microbiome isn't flourishing, and the gut and brain are not functioning optimally.

HEAL YOUR GUT ...

HEAL YOUR BRAIN

WHY A HEALTHY GUT IS CRUCIAL FOR STROKE RECOVERY

Eighty percent of our body's first line of defense – our immune system – is in our gut lining. For this reason, nurturing a healthy gut is crucial during stroke recovery and the rest of your life because it can help prevent a second stroke.

Can A Healthy Gut Help to Relieve Depression & Heal Your Brain?

There are many studies that link an unhealthy microbiome to anxiety and depression. One explanation for this is that your microbiome assists with the production of GABA, a neurotransmitter that's known for improving mood and relieving anxiety. A healthy microbiome also helps reduce cortisol levels – the stress hormone. So, a happy gut not only boosts your mood, but it also helps counteract the negative effects of stress. A healthy microbiome is absolutely essential for a healthy mood and a healthy recovery.

- 80% of our immune system is in our gut.

- There are more nerves in our gut than our brain.

- Our gut influences our brain, heart & mood.

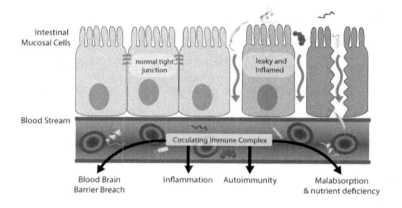

Learn More @ www.ionbiome.com

CELLULAR HEALTH

Our bodies are constantly bombarded with toxins from our environment, from the air we breathe to the food we eat. Even our largest organ, our skin, is invaded by skin care products and lotions that are filled with chemicals that tear down our immune system. All these play havoc on our ability to heal. In addition to proper nutrition, we need good supplements in order to boost and restore our system.

It's an unfortunate fact that our own "civilized" food supply no longer feeds us well nutritionally. Our food is comforting and tastes good, but as far as our cells are concerned, too much of what we eat is over-processed, denatured and acidic, and ends up depleting our bodies— robbing us rather than feeding us. Today's western diet has double the caloric intake of a consumer in 1965, and we are receiving seventy-five percent less nutrient value for current calories consumed. Seeking daily, quality nutrient supplementation is no longer an option but a requirement for health. We all need to supplement our diets in the most efficient and economical means possible.

Like most of us, I don't enjoy taking lots of supplements. Not only can it be expensive, having them all work together in synergy is not often easy. So, I was directed by experts to an advanced multi-vitamin that has an all-in-one system.

The one I selected has ninety plus vitamins, minerals, and protective phytonutrients, combined with probiotics and enzymes for advanced cellular nutrition. It includes AM and PM formulas for a 24-hour cycle of nutrition, phytonutrients for different aspects of cell health, and absorption boosting ingredients. It also includes specific phytonutrients that have been shown to have positive effects at the cellular level.

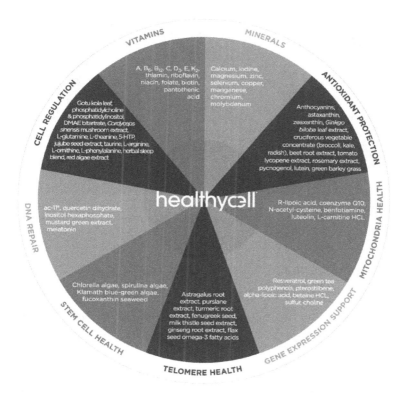

For those who do not like taking pills, they also have a liquid gel form that can be easily mixed in water or put in a smoothie. Learn more @ www.HealthyCell.com

TURMERIC

Turmeric is one of the healthiest spices on Earth. Research shows that it could be beneficial to stroke patients by encouraging new cells to grow and preventing cell death after a stroke.

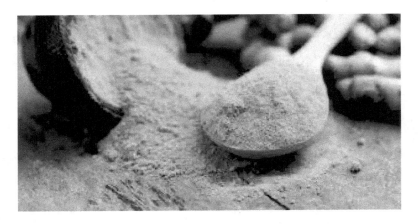

Turmeric is a safe, powerful, inflammation-fighting superstar that has been used for thousands of years in Ayurvedic and Traditional Chinese Medicine. It is one the most thoroughly researched plants in existence today. Its medicinal properties and components (primarily curcumin) have been the subject of over 12,000 peer-reviewed and published biomedical studies. In fact, this sacred plant has revealed over 800 potential preventive and therapeutic applications, as well as 250 distinct beneficial physiological effects. The list of curcumin's preventive and healing properties is a long one.

According to a study conducted at M.D. Anderson Cancer Center's Department of Experimental Therapeutics:

"Curcumin has been shown to exhibit antioxidant, anti-inflammatory, antiviral, antibacterial, antifungal, and anticancer activities and thus has a really significant potential effect against various malignant diseases, diabetes, allergies, arthritis, Alzheimer's disease, and other chronic illnesses."

Like everything else, quality is key. Not all turmeric is equal. Many of the turmeric/curcumin supplements today potentially provide very little benefit to your body, if any at all. So, be very selective.

REFLEXOLOGY

Reflexology is a natural healing art. It is based on the principle that there are reflexes in the hands and feet that correspond to every part, gland and organ of the body. Through application of pressure on these reflexes, reflexology relieves tension, improves circulation and promotes the natural function of the related areas of the body. Reflexology encourages greater relaxation and increases the overall effectiveness of the body's ability to heal. It has been used to assist stroke rehabilitation by improving circulation and helping to adjust body imbalances. The use of this gentle treatment supports those recovering from stroke and enhances overall well-being.

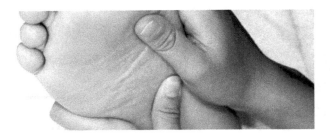

When I was in the hospital following my stroke, a dear friend of my family who was a reflexologist would treat me while visiting me. She worked on the big toe of my affected side. It was sore but felt so good, and after a few minutes the soreness was gone. Little did I know at the time that this was pushing blood back up to my brain, an ancient form of healing. Ever since, I have sessions as often as possible and have seen it help a lot of my people.

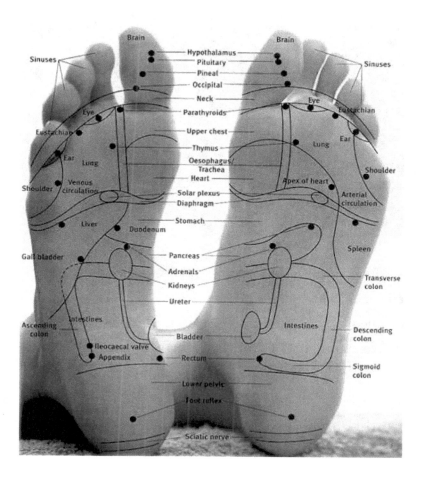

Brain
Sinuses
Hypothalamus
Pituitary
Pineal
Occipital
Neck
Eye
Parathyroids
Upper chest
Eustachian
Ear
Thymus
Lung
Oesophagus/
Trachea
Heart
Venous
Apex of heart
Shoulder
circulation
Solar plexus
Shoulder
Diaphragm
Arterial
circulation
Liver
Stomach
Duodenum
Spleen
Gall bladder
Pancreas
Adrenals
Kidneys
Transverse
colon
Ureter
Ascending
colon
Intestines
Intestines
Descending
colon
Ileocaecal valve
Bladder
Appendix
Rectum
Sigmoid
colon
Lower pelvic
Foot reflex
Sciatic nerve

Brain
Sinuses
Eye
Eustachian
Lung
Ear

ESSENTIAL OILS

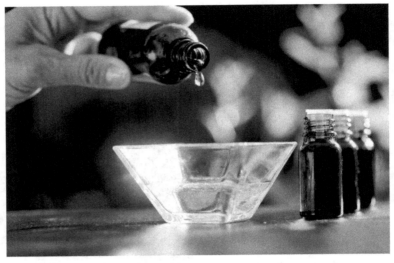

Pure therapeutic grade essential oils can be very beneficial for the brain and stroke recovery. Essential oils are distilled from various parts of plants, including seeds, bark, leaves, stems, roots, flowers and fruit. The essential oils of the plant help fight infection and initiate regeneration. They possess potent anti-bacterial, antifungal and anti-viral properties. The molecules of essential oils are also relatively small, giving them the ability to easily penetrate the cells, and some oils have been shown to cross the blood-brain barrier. When topically applied to the feet or elsewhere, essential oils can travel throughout the body in a matter of minutes.

Quality Matters

Many oils on the market shelves today are produced using chemicals and high heat. It is imperative to only use high-quality therapeutic grade essential oils distilled at low heat, without chemicals and pesticide free. Fragrance oils or chemical components of essential oils produced in a lab bring disappointing results and may even be toxic. My personal choice is www.YoungLiving.com. Some of my favorite oils are Frankincense, Brain Power, and Rosemary.

CRANIOSACRAL THERAPY

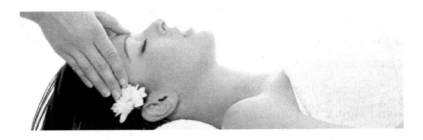

CranioSacral Therapy (CST) can support the healing and recovery process after a stroke. CST is a very gentle, hands-on method of evaluating and enhancing the functioning of a physiological body system called the craniosacral system - comprised of the membranes and cerebrospinal fluid that surround and protect the brain and spinal cord. CST helps to improve the nervous system and eliminate deeply held traumas, such as a stroke. Like the pulse of the cardiovascular system, the CranioSacral system has a rhythm that can be felt throughout the body. Using a very light touch, skilled practitioners can monitor this rhythm at key body areas to pinpoint the source of an obstruction or stress. The treatment itself involves the application of very light forces applied by the therapist's hands. Limbs may be picked up and moved gently and slowly as the body tissues are allowed to "unwind" themselves. A typical session lasts an hour. Its far-reaching effects enable CranioSacral Therapy to be useful for a wide scope of health problems, including stroke. Again, be selective of your practitioner. I only select a therapist trained in the original techniques of Dr. John Upledger, an osteopathic physician and surgeon. www.upledger.com

MASSAGE THERAPY

Scientific studies have shown that when massaged, stroke survivors experienced increased mobility, decreased pain, decreased depression, and as a result used less medication. Massage provides ten times as much oxygen to the massaged areas as the body would receive passively in fifteen minutes. Circulating blood is the great communicator and supplier of essentials, and as long as blood is freely circulating, there is healing going on.

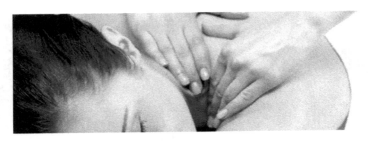

Massage in Stroke Patients Have Been Shown To:

- Improve Mobility

- Relieve Fatigue

- Help Insomnia

- Improve Circulation

- Decrease Pain and Cramps

- Alleviate Symptoms of Depression

Aquatic Therapy

Aquatic therapy (pool therapy) is used as a treatment modality in the rehabilitation process. It is physical therapy that is performed in the water using buoyant Styrofoam weights along with other exercises. Some pools even have an underwater treadmill. For a stroke survivor, aquatic therapy is especially helpful as the water removes the limitations of gravity, providing the ability to do more in the pool than on land and ultimately achieving therapeutic goals quicker.

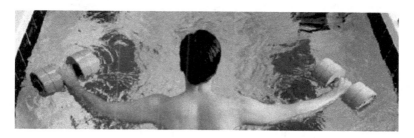

Pool activities include stretches and strengthening, balance and coordination, walking and aerobics. I prefer to use an outdoor pool or one that is not chlorinated as chlorine can weaken the immune system. Also, you might want to wear rubber booties to protect the bottom of your feet while you step vigorously against the concrete bottom.

Regenerative Sleep

Sleep plays a vital role in healing and repair of our heart and blood vessels. Ongoing sleep deficiency is linked to an increased risk of heart disease, kidney disease, high blood pressure, diabetes, and stroke. In those who suffered a stroke, the regulatory centers have been compromised and must be rebuilt. The brain needs to rest from all the physical work of creating new neural pathways. The only solution is to sleep.

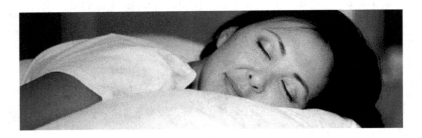

Sleep is Still the Best Medicine

- Sleeping a lot after a stroke is perfectly normal and necessary.

- Sleep cleans the brain from damaging toxins.

- Sleep is #1 for stroke rehabilitation.

- Sleep helps your memory.

- Sleep helps the brain repair and rewire itself.

Broad-Spectrum Hemp-Derived CBD Oil

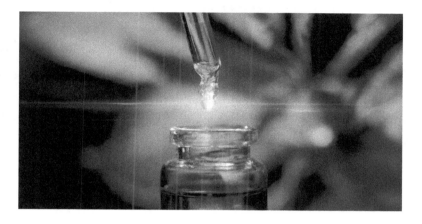

**Recover faster, sleep better,
calm the mind, and reduce pain.**

CBD is a non-psychoactive component extracted from the hemp plant. It has a wide range of therapeutic benefits. Even though CBD and THC are from the same plant species, they have distinct properties that separate them from one another. THC is associated with the high feeling or psychoactive effects, and CBD is more well known for its health benefits. CBD works with your body's natural rhythms to increase focus and reduce anxiety by increasing serotonin levels in the brain. Even better, CBD does not have intoxicating properties like THC, and it won't cause drowsiness or make you sleepy during the day. It can actually help you be more alert and productive and then shut down a racing mind in the evening to get better sleep.

Broad-Spectrum CBD contains most of the compounds found in full-spectrum CBD—except for THC.

While full-spectrum extracts can contain up to 0.3% THC, broad-spectrum oils don't have any measurable amount of it. Another benefit is known as the "entourage effect." What this means is that the very combination of many compounds (less THC) boosts each individual therapeutic ability at once. This may help protect stroke patients from brain damage and even aid recovery by boosting brain function. Broad-Spectrum CBD generally costs more than CBD, but I have found it to be worth the difference.

HOW DOES CBD WORK?

The key to CBD health benefits is the Endocannabinoid system (ECS) - a network of receptors in the cells. The system is there to maintain homeostasis (balance) within the body. In response to toxins in our body, it releases cannabinoids to set things back to their natural state. Some of the systems that the ECS helps to balance are mood, sleep, memory, temperature regulation, pain, appetite, digestion, immune function, inflammation, and motor control. So, basically, just about everything. It's really an amazing God-given system that's been completely overlooked.

Over time, with aging, the endocannabinoid system eventually burns out. Fewer cannabinoids are released, so the body's levels deplete. CBD oil can boost your endocannabinoid system – relieving aches and pains, improving sleep cycles, mood, memory, focus, and more. And the best part is, there are no psychoactive effects, so you get relief without any "high,"

The most common and effective way that CBD oil is consumed is through sublingual administration. This is when you place a few drops of the oil under your tongue. You should hold these drops under your tongue for up to 30 seconds. This gives the oil enough time to diffuse into your bloodstream through the tissues in your tongue. CBD is only effective when it enters the bloodstream. The more CBD you can get into the bloodstream, the more effective it is likely to be.

There are many brands and sources being promoted so be selective. Many CBD oil products are poorly processed and may be tainted with toxic solvent residues, pesticides, corn syrup, artificial flavors and colors, and other contaminants. The key things I look for are: 100% organic, Broad-Spectrum, quickly absorbed and taste good. My personal choice is www.PureCBDExtraStrength.com

GROUNDING

The most primitive, easiest, and cheapest way to create optimal health, even after a stroke, is Grounding or Earthing, as it is often called. This simply means connecting to the Earth's natural, negative surface charge by being barefoot outside- a simple concept, but one with profound impact on the physiology.

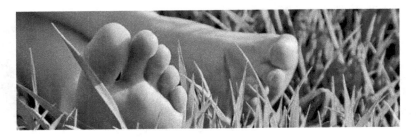

According to Stephen Sinatra, MD, a board-certified cardiologist, "when you ground to the electron-enriched earth, an improved balance of the sympathetic and parasympathetic nervous system occurs."

The Earthing Institute states;

"Connection with the Earth restores a lost electrical signal to the body that seems to stabilize the complicated circuitry of our essentially-electrical body. Our built-in self-regulating and self-healing mechanisms become more effective. There are head-to-toe improvements. Better blood flow. Less pain and inflammation. More energy. Deeper sleep."

For me, I will either walk barefooted in a maintained grassy area (no ant piles or poop) or sit in a chair while placing my feet on the ground. A little moisture is always beneficial, like the dew in the morning or the water's edge at the beach. Perhaps that is why we feel so good after a walk on the beach.

Benefits:

According to emerging research, Earthing can be beneficial in:

- Reducing inflammation by defusing excess positive electrons
- Reducing chronic pain
- Improving Sleep
- Increasing Energy
- Lowering stress and promoting calmness by reducing stress hormones.
- Normalizing biological rhythms including circadian rhythm
- Improving blood pressure and blood flow
- Relieving muscle tension and headache
- Lessens menstrual and female hormone symptoms
- Speeds healing- used in some places to prevent bed sores
- Can eliminate jet lag
- Protecting the body from EMFs
- Shortens recovery time from injury or athletic activity
- Reducing or eliminating snoring
- Helping support adrenal health

ACUPUNCTURE

Acupuncture therapy for stroke-caused conditions such as paralysis, speech and swallowing problems, and depression is commonly used in the Orient. In China and Japan, an acupuncturist is likely to start therapy as soon as possible after a stroke. Many studies have been conducted on the effects of acupuncture during stroke rehabilitation. These studies show that acupuncture reduces hospital stays and improves recovery speed. Acupuncture has been shown to help stroke patients regain motor and cognitive skills and to improve their ability to manage daily functioning. These therapies work with the natural vital energy inherent within all living things to promote the body's ability to heal itself.

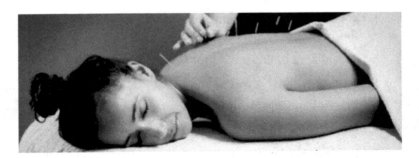

Like most of us, I do not like needles. Just the thought of having a bunch of them stuck in me makes my hair stand up. But I was pleasantly surprised to find the acupuncture sessions to be painless and relaxing, especially when the heat light was applied. Would you believe I actually fell asleep?

ATLAS ORTHOGONAL

The Atlas Orthogonal system is a painless and safe spinal correction which restores body balance and increases the body's natural healing ability. Because of the precise measurements and X-ray analysis, a correction can be made without any forceful movements or twisting of the neck or back.

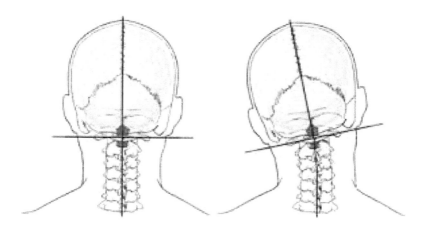

The Atlas – or C1 is the guide and protector for the brain stem and spinal cord. The spinal cord and brainstem pass through the atlas and communicate with the rest of the body. The vertebral arteries pass through the sides of the Atlas and supply the back third of the brain with blood. When in alignment, there is little to no stress to the joints and discs below. There is no nerve irrigation, and there is normal blood flow through the vertebral arteries to the brain and brain-stem.

The Atlas guides the master network of the body – the nervous system. It supports the skull and is considered by many as the most important vertebrae.

Everyone should have this checked, especially after a trauma like a stroke.

STEM CELL THERAPY

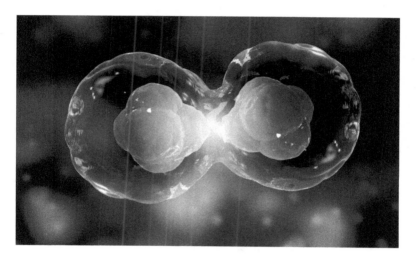

A stem cell is a "generic" cell that can make exact copies of itself indefinitely. In addition, a stem cell has the ability to produce specialized cells for various tissues in the body — such as heart muscle, brain tissue, and liver tissue. "Stem-cell therapy offers the potential to bring back some motor function," says Dr. Leonid Groysman, associate professor of neurology at UCI School of Medicine.

I received a series of stem cells. After years passed, an obvious benefit that was visible to everyone was that I had not aged, which isn't a bad thing, but an expensive fountain of youth. Don't get me wrong, stem cell therapy certainly has its place and can fuel the recovery process, I just prefer to try everything else first.

Fortunately, there are ways your body can produce its own stem cells. So before rushing out to receive a series of costly injections, I would encourage you to strengthen and build up your body first and then reassess. Either way, always do your research on the clinic; the method of procedure; origin of the cells and how they were harvested. Not all are equal, and some can be unsafe.

LAUGHTER

Laughter is medicine for the soul, and it's free to all. Patients, doctors and health-care professionals are all finding that laughter may indeed be the best medicine. Hospitals around the world are incorporating formal and informal laughter therapy programs into their therapeutic regimens.

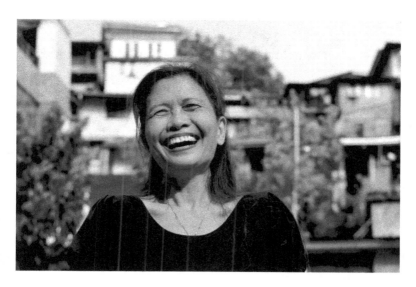

Laughter increases circulation and improves the delivery of oxygen and nutrients to tissues throughout your body. Laughter is a natural healer. Over the years, many physical benefits to laughter have been reported by doctors and health care professionals.

- Decrease in stress hormone levels

- Strengthening of the immune system

- Muscle relaxation

- Pain reduction

- Lowering of blood pressure

- Cardiovascular conditioning

- Natural anti-depression

Whether watching a comedy, playing with your kids or pets, or cutting up with a friend, take a "time out" from being so serious and make it a point to laugh every single day.

PRAYER

Prayer is shown to have a profound effect on our health. Research has shown that spiritual healing can provide permanent relief from the worries and difficulties that plague us. It can bring us about a complete revolution in the consciousness and the body. It can affect enduring physical, mental, and emotional change. A community of faith can provide more than support when we are in need of help. The members of a faith community can strengthen our resolve to heal, can link their prayers to ours, and can restore us to faith. They can envelop us in caring and love. There's no debating the power of prayer and its transformative impact in the lives of people throughout the world and throughout history.

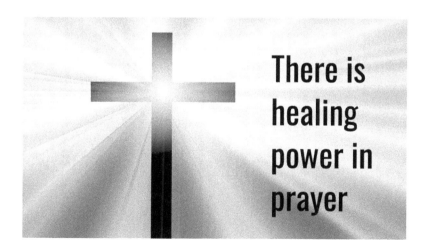

There is healing power in prayer

My recovery was covered with many prayers, and God blessed me with messengers to show me the way. Now all my days begin with a prayer. I discovered that prayers are simply conversations with God. My conversations with Him are like talking with a good friend. At times, I think I make Him laugh.

Stress Management

When people are stressed out, they often say, "I just can't think right now." That's because stress increases the amount of cortisol produced in the adrenal glands and raised cortisol levels restrict the flow of oxygen to the brain. It may explain why a lot of strokes happen on Monday's, holidays, and at times when people go through grief or major loss. From normal challenges to major crises, stress is part of life. And while you can't always control your circumstances, you can control how you respond to them.

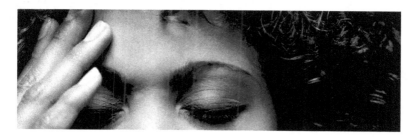

There are many techniques that will help to relieve stress. Some of the simplest forms I have found to be very effective both during my recovery, and now, are to:

- Find a change of scenery, somewhere with trees or water.

- Put my bare feet on grass.

- Express all the things I am grateful for.

- Breathe. Just changing the way you breathe can make a big difference to your overall stress level. Breathe in through your nose and imagine that you're inhaling peaceful, calm air. Breathing techniques can calm your body and your brain in just a few minutes.

- Hug. When you hug someone, oxytocin is released. Oxytocin also causes a reduction in blood pressure. It reduces the stress hormone norepinephrine and can produce a sense of relaxation.

IMPROVING BALANCE & STABILITY

After a stroke, most of us are challenged with balance and stability. During a trade show, I was shown a product that is simple and quite amazing. The best of modern technology with decades of research in neuromuscular science - drug-free and without invasive treatments.

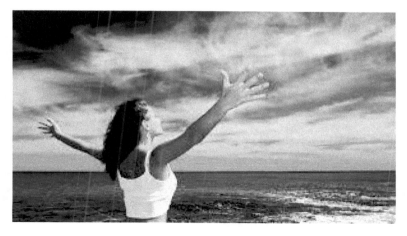

It starts with a special tactile pattern known as VOXX HPT. This pattern is specially woven into socks and insoles. When you wear either the socks, insoles, or patches, contact with the Voxx HPT pattern triggers a neuro response that sends information from the receptors on the bottom of your feet (or the inside of your forearm) to your brainstem that helps manage pain, as well as improve mobility and balance.

After processing that information, the Central Nervous System (CNS) distributes commands to your peripheral nervous system, affecting various functions in your body, from pain regulation to motor control and balance. The effect is instant, ranging from improved balance, mobility and pain management to better energy level and recovery process. Learn more @ www.VoxxLife.com.

INDOOR AIR QUALITY

Now more than ever people are looking for safe yet powerful solutions to purify the air and surfaces in their home. We cannot avoid pollution outside, but we can when we are indoors. – where we spend most of our lives. When we breathe, pollutants get into our lungs; they can enter the bloodstream and be carried to our internal organs such as the brain.

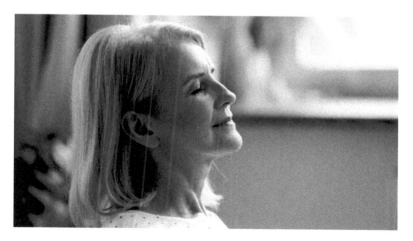

If the COVID-19 pandemic taught us anything, it's that air borne viruses are real and can endanger our lives and well-being. To protect ourselves, we must strengthen our immune system with good nutrients like Vitamin C, D3, and Zinc; drink clean water; and breathe clean air.

Once again, advanced technology provides a way to treat the air and surfaces in your home on a continuous basis. But not all purifiers are the same. The system that I personally use is based on a technology originally developed by NASA. It is perhaps the most powerful air and surface purification technology ever discovered. This Certified Space Technology safely eliminates 99.9 percent of airborne and surface bacteria, viruses, mold, fungus, & Volatile Organic Compounds (VOCs) such as cleaning products, paints, and disinfecting products. It has been tested on SARS-cov-2 virus (which is the cause of COVID) and has been scientifically proven to kill the virus. Learn more @www.ActivePure.com.

OLD WAY - NEW WAY

For decades, well-meaning people have prescribed the same outline for recovery. But, if you're willing to investigate a new way that most people don't know to tell you, your life can be transformed.

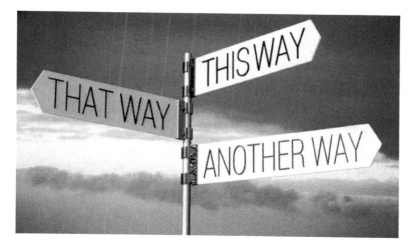

Old Way

- Go to rehab forever
- Take lots of medications
- Undergo risky & often very expensive procedures.
- Avoid certain foods and activities
- Wear braces that often require altering shoes
- Accept limitations as the new normal
- On and on ...

New Way

- Renew Your Mind – Your Master Key
- Use the Integrative Approach - "Your Secret Weapons"
- Be consistent and Never Give Up

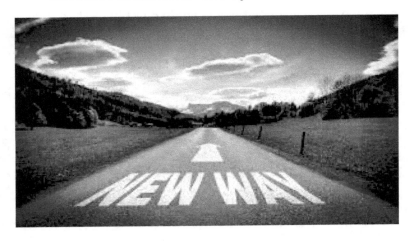

CASE STUDY #2

MARK. PROFESSIONAL BUSINESSMAN. AGE 65

Mark is a businessman who suffered a massive stroke. When I met him, he had lost his self-confidence, motivation and enthusiasm for living. He had tried everything, and nothing seemed to provide results. He realized he needed a coach to provide direction and empowerment. I customized a program for him and taught him how to properly utilize his "secret weapons." After six months he told me for the first time in over ten years he felt like a new man. He started a new business and is thriving both physically and emotionally. He even started dating and plans to remarry.

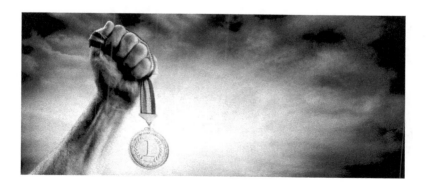

THE WAY OF THE WARRIOR

Quick Recap

At this point we know that to win the battle and overcome we must have:

1. A positive faith filled mindset

2. Awareness

3. The right tools

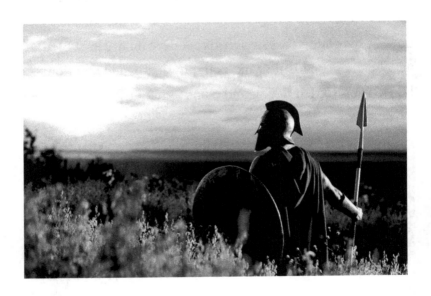

KEY #4

FIND YOUR WHY

Leverage Your Determination

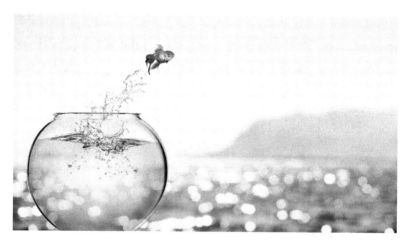

Most of us have at some time in our life have experienced feeling a supernatural strength and determination when we were suddenly propelled to act, like when we witness a loved one being harmed or in need. I've heard stories of people lifting a car seeing their child stuck under it. Or when you work extra overtime to buy a special gift for someone you love. That's the grit I'm talking about. Find it and use it. Pray and ask for it. God knows we only can only do so much on our own. This life is more than any of us can handle on our own.

It has been said that difficulties don't determine who we are, rather they REVEAL who we are. Said another way, what's in us usually comes out when we are squeezed. When your back is against the wall this is when you will see what you are all about.

We all have days that are harder than others. You'll hit rough patches along the trail up your mountain. This is normal. Just never forget that in order to get *through* something - <u>you must keep going.</u> Stopping to wallow in despair or depression will only delay your victory. Take a break and eat something good, reach out to a neighbor or friend, get dressed and get out. Just NEVER ever give up! Your victory awaits!

- Be determined on purpose.
- To thyself be true and to all those you love and that love you.
- Your spouse, children, companion, and family need you.
- Your life was spared for a reason and it's no accident you're reading this.

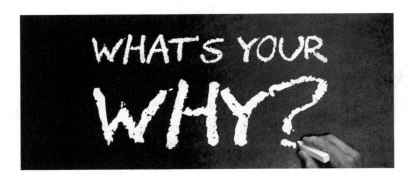

Case Study #3

CATHY. CAREGIVER FOR SON. MASSIVE STROKE. AGE 19

Cathy's son went to bed complaining of a bad headache after being hit in the head playing sports. He woke the next morning paralyzed and unable to speak. At the age of nineteen his life took a dramatic turn. For years, both he and his determined mother went everywhere and did anything to help him. After exhausting all their efforts, she reached out for my help. I have to say it was a tough case, but I started with his mindset and even though he was unable to speak, I insisted on talking with him via zoom so we could see one another. He would smile as I talked about his dreams and goals. Little by little he started showing signs of improvement. He even uttered "Mom."

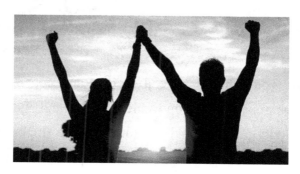

KEY #5

ASK FOR HELP

Take Action

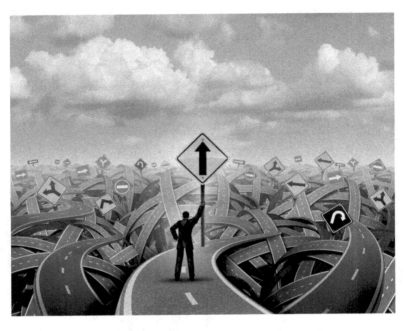

Everyone should have a mentor and coach, someone who has gone before you to clear a path and show you the way. Good guidance and mentoring are so important. Having a coach with a roadmap will not only help you reach your goals faster; you can avoid costly mistakes and be encouraged to keep moving forward. Find a mentor who is where you want to go and learn from their experience.

It is my hope that every stroke survivor will discover the keys to overcome as I did. First and foremost, you must ask God for help.

Ask and it will be given to you; seek and you will find; knock, and the door will be opened to you. - Matt 7:7 (NIV)

Life is challenging, and we all need help – especially after a stroke. I knew overcoming this would require greater help than my family, friends or doctors could provide. Deep down I knew it was something only God could fix. I had known about Him all my life but had never really asked for His help. Now, I needed Him more than ever. These days you might not hear God or Jesus used much as it is often replaced with general terms like "Universe" or "Energy," and while He is all that, it is important to know Him by name. Jesus is the son of the living God who came to Earth to die for us so we might have eternal life. The most famous verse in the Bible says it all ...

For God so loved the world that he gave his one and only Son, that whoever believes in him shall not perish but have eternal life. - John 3:16 (NIV)

I recently saw a T-shirt that read: J E S U S is the password to heaven. We all know how important a password is to access anything of value. Since God tells us that the only way to get to Him is through His Son Jesus, then it's important to know His name and to use it. Simply call out to Him and ask Him to save you. He will hear you and never leave you.

Let not your heart be troubled: ye believe in God, believe also in me. In my Father's house are many mansions: if it were not so, I would have told you. I go to prepare a place for you. And if I go and prepare a place for you, I will come again, and receive you unto myself; that where I am, there ye may be also. - John 14:1-3 (KJV)

Having faith gives you an anchor in the storms of this life. I can't imagine how I would have survived without it. Faith gave me strength and courage to press on, and still does. Faith is believing in miracles and possibilities without seeing them first. It's knowing that with God on your side, nothing is impossible. Once you believe that, everything changes. You will never be the same. You will not fear the future or worry about how things will work out (unless you choose to). It's perfectly natural to be afraid, but God will give you strength and courage. So, when there seems to be no way, and you've done all you can do, you must let go and trust God to take over. He is your way maker and can move mountains! He can do what medicine cannot. He is the great physician and healer. You can rest because He will not!

I've been told I have a lot of faith, but you don't need

great faith. Jesus used the tiniest seed to describe how the faith of a mustard seed can move mountains. Stroke was my mountain, but I chose to believe that with God's help I would overcome it. Yes, it took time, and it was by no means a cake walk, but I trusted God to guide me and show me the way. He was beside me the entire time and brought me safely through to recovery. So, take hope my friend - God is in control and has a good plan. You wouldn't be breathing if God didn't have something great prepared. Stay encouraged. Restoration is coming!

As you set out on your journey, I have to forewarn you about an enemy that is very real - one that is often overlooked as a religious myth. You've probably heard him loosely depicted as a cartoon character - a red man with horns and a pitchfork, but he is far from it. He is beautiful, charming, and incredibly deceptive. He will even disguise himself as an angel of light. Once an angel named Lucifer, he was cast out of heaven to hades (another word for hell) and is the prince of darkness, king of evil, and father of lies known as Satan. He is compared to a lurking lion seeking whom he may devour. His goal is to take us down with him. He will lie to you and tell you that you've reached your limit, that you can't overcome; he will try to make you think you are disqualified, incapable and hopeless. All lies. Fear and anxiety are two of his greatest weapons he will use against us. He creates doubt, despair, and division. I'm telling you all this because you've got to be prepared to combat the anxiety and fear he will use to trick your mind and cloud your vision. You've got to know how to recognize his schemes and defeat his deception. Remember, the "darkness" hates the "light" or said differently, evil hates good. If you've ever watched any vampire movies you will recall that just as the Count was ready to attack a person, a cross was held up to repel him. Today, I think of the enemy like a vampire – seeking to suck the life out of us by stealing our peace, hope, and joy. Sometimes it is subtle, and we don't realize it until his fangs start to bite. My power over him comes when I remind him who I am and whose I am – a child of the most-high God. It's like holding up a cross to a vampire and opening a window to let the sun burst in. God is far more powerful and only He has the final say.

We are living in unprecedented times. Our world is in a serious time of turmoil and spiraling out of control. Personally, I believe we are living out the final Bible prophecies and we will see Christ's return within our lifetime. The signs are all around us. Never before in history have current events been so aligned with End Times' prophecy. While no man can know the day or time, we must be ready. He will come in a blink of an eye when we are least expected and rapture all those who believe in Him. It could be anytime – today, tomorrow, or next year. Either way, He IS coming back and the most important decision you will ever make in this life is knowing where you will spend the next for all eternity. As your fellow stroke survivor, I urge you to be sure of this one thing - know where you will spend eternity. There are only two destinations and I want to see all of you at the pearly gates. I'm sure a lot of people will dismiss this as nonsense - but it's not. As one teacher says ... *"if I'm wrong about all this it's no big deal, but if you're wrong, it's a REALLY BIG DEAL!"* Heed the warning. Believe and accept His invitation to eternal life and receive Him as your Savior. It's a free gift that can't be bought or earned. Simply ask Jesus to save and help you. He wants to give you a breakthrough. It may not happen on your timetable or as you expect. It may not be logical or make sense. So be diligent and prepared so you may be able to discern when it does arrive. Faith will light your way. Taking action will move you forward to the things God has in store. Just know you are never alone. Jesus loves you and will see you through.

So do not fear,
for I am with you;
do not be dismayed,
for I am your God.
I will **strengthen** you
and **help** you;
I will **uphold** you with
my righteous right hand.

-Isaiah 41:10

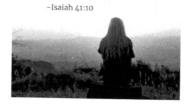

I'll close with a well-known story ...

There once was a man who lived in a two-story house. The house was near a river and unfortunately the river began to flood.

As the river rose, warnings were given via radio, TV, and shortwave. Large jeeps drove through the area to evacuate people. As a jeep drove by the man's house, he was told:

"You are in danger. Your life is at stake. You must evacuate. Get in the Jeep. Let us help you evacuate."

"No," the man replied from his doorstep. "I have faith. I will be okay. The flood won't get me. God will take care of me."

The water continued to rise.

Soon the man was on the second floor. A boat was going through the area and arrived at the man's house. Rescuers made every effort to convince the man to take action so that his life would be saved.

"You are in danger. Your life is at stake. You will drown in the flood."

"No worries," says the man. "I have faith. Everything is okay. Even though the flood is rising, I will be fine. God will take care of me."

The flood continued to rise.

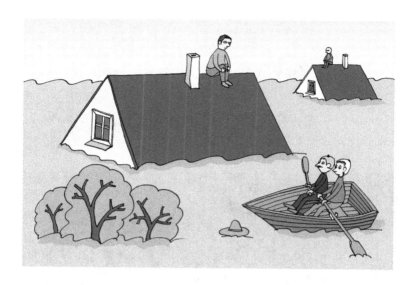

The man went to the roof to avoid the rising water. A helicopter pilot sees him on top of the roof and hovers above the man. Using a megaphone, the pilot tries to convince the man to grab the rope ladder which was dangling above his head

"You are in danger. The flood is still rising. You will drown if you do not grab the rope ladder. Let us help you."

"No worries." says the man. "I will be fine. Yes, the flood is higher, but I have faith. God will take care of me."

The flood rises. The man drowns.

At the pearly gates, the man says to God, "Why didn't you help me?"

To which God replies: "I sent you a jeep, a boat, and a helicopter."

Faith Without Action Is Dead

Be Ready to Take Action!

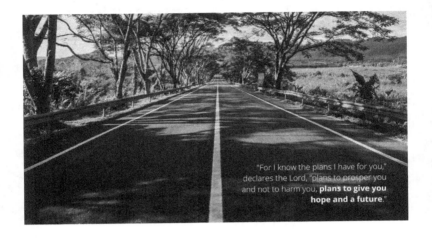

"For I know the plans I have for you," declares the Lord, "plans to prosper you and not to harm you, **plans to give you hope and a future**."

CONCLUSION

Get your hopes up! Regeneration and healing after a stroke are possible. I'm living proof! With over twenty years of personal experience, it has been a blessing to help stroke survivors around the world. It is my heart's desire to use my personal experience to empower and help you discover answers and solutions and to fill your heart with hope. I have been where you are and understand your challenges. It's time to take action and set yourself free. There has never been a better time with more amazing treatments, products and ideas that can accelerate recovery and improve your quality of life. Get up, take action and finish the race set before you! Having a stroke is not how your story ends.

"And now may the Lord bless you, and may the Lord keep you; may the Lord make His face to shine upon you. May the Lord be gracious unto you and give you His peace.

With Faith, Hope & Love,

Author, Speaker & Overcomer
America's Stroke Coach
www.ValerieGreene.com
888-942-9355

ABOUT THE AUTHOR

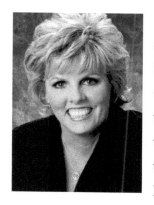 As an internationally recognized stroke advocate and compassionate leader in stroke awareness, Valerie Greene has inspired audiences around the world. At age thirty-one, Valerie was a healthy, vibrant businesswoman until a massive stroke paralyzed the left side of her body and left her unable to speak. Doctors told her that she might never walk or talk again, and most of her hearing was lost. Sheer determination and faith propelled her out of her wheelchair and into a new life learning once more how to walk and communicate. Now a worldwide symbol of hope, Valerie has become a beacon of light to millions. Founder and CEO of Global Stroke Resource and B-Center, Inc. she is a published author and speaker. Valerie has appeared on CBS, NBC, ABC and FOX raising public awareness of stroke prevention and recovery. Through nearly two decades of her recovery odyssey, Valerie has gathered a collection of treatments and fundamentals to assist the body's ability to regenerate and heal. Her passion and life purpose are to help others through stroke while letting them know that they are not alone and to NEVER give up.

CPSIA information can be obtained
at www.ICGtesting.com
Printed in the USA
BVHW041309291221
625055BV00018B/1670